DR. RONSPEAKS

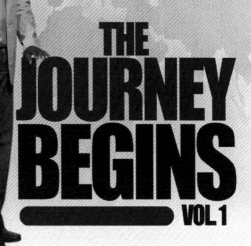

THE
JOURNEY
BEGINS

VOL 1

Dr. Rondrick Williamson

Editor: Shann Hall- LochmannVanBennekom

Cover Adjuster: Rob King

Layout Designer: Ileta Randall

Graphic Designer: Edd Anderson

Photographers: Keith Hammock (front cover) and Donald Crenshaw (back cover)

ISBN: 978-1-938950-28-5

Greater Is He Publishing Company

9824 E. Washington St.

Chagrin Falls, Ohio 44023

Mailing Address:

P O. Box 46115 Bedford, Ohio 44146

Office 216.288.9315

Purchase Books Online
at www.GreaterIsHePublishing.com

Acknowledgment

This book has evolved over many years. It is important for me to recognize those key persons who were instrumental in the process. Thank you to the following individuals who without their contributions and support this book would not have been written: my mother Carrie Thomas and my two brothers Terrance and Mario. They helped me to realize I had something special deep inside of me. Hats off also to a host of family and loved ones who carried the torch even during times when I grew weary and discouraged. To my special friend, Cynthia Linguard you will always hold a very warm place in my heart. Thank you for being a true friend through the ups and downs.

TABLE OF CONTENTS

Chapter 1
Every Step

"Every step on the stairway of life has its lessons to be learned. The key is to learn as much as you can and keep climbing."

Do you ever wonder how to keep walking when it seems as if your terrain is sinking sand? How do you see the light at the end of the tunnel when there is no hope? These are the dark places that life affords us if we just keep living. What do you do when life deals you a bad hand? Certainly the day will come. No one is exempt from this, not even me. My life certainly has not been a utopia—that ideal place of perfectness. If I must say, it's been exactly the opposite.

Questions then arise. Do you allow your present location to determine your future destination? What is more important to you? I guess one could say, "Well, I'm here, so why not just continue to live the life that was given me?" That's settling. The alternative would be to endeavor to be better than your current situation. That's striving. Which category do you place yourself?

"Settlers" find their current situation both adequate and sufficient. Their comfort level blinds them to the opportunities that may await them, should they put forth a small amount of effort. They become a slave to their surroundings.

The "striver," however, is never comfortable with mediocrity. He or she sees life as a canvas of unfinished business. I'm a "striver." Having lived in a single-parent home with my mother and my two younger brothers, we faced the reality of the "have nots." The "settling" and "striving" mentalities are all too familiar to me. We were not at the point of privation, however. We had the basic necessities of life: food, water, shelter, and clothing. The most important thing we had was each other. Of course, hindsight is always 20/20. As most children did, we wanted the newest and latest trends in fashion: the Members Only jacket, the parachute pants, and the stone washed jeans. All of the popular kids wore these styles.

> "The simple things in life are often overlooked. But often times, they are the most important."

Yes, we struggled to make it. My mom was the bread winner. I don't remember my biological father ever being in the home. He and my mother married and divorced soon after I was born. Looking back at my early childhood years, any memories I have of him are vague. Both of my parents were teenagers when I was conceived. I think the marriage occurred because of pressure from my maternal grandmother. At that time, having a child out of wedlock was considered taboo. I guess it didn't matter whether or not the

Chapter 1 Every Step

two parties loved each other; marriage was a given. So they married, and, of course, it didn't last. The divorce was bitter, and at the time, my mother found out she was expecting a second child. Of course, my dad denied that he was the father of this child. He accused my mom of infidelity. I guess this was his way of not having to take care of another kid. My mom knew, without a doubt, that this new baby was his. He did a great job of convincing his family and the courts that she was allegedly lying and having an extramarital affair. This was hurtful, demeaning, and devastating to my mom who was just barely out of high school. The court case was not really one at all.

My mother and her family couldn't afford an attorney for adequate representation, but my father was able to. Case closed. We all know how that ended.

When some people have a little cash on hand, they can make things happen—even if it's not the truth. Several years after my brother Terrance was born, my mom birthed

my second sibling, Mario. He was a bundle of joy. We were

like three peas in a pod. We loved the camera. We would

take turns, one would be the photographer, the other two

his subjects.

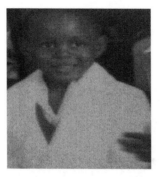

Mom did the best she could to provide the finest life

for us. My grandmother assisted whenever and wherever

she could. We even lived with her for a while. She was a

strong-willed, church-going woman, and was the matriarch

of our family. Her husband had passed years prior from a

heart attack. I wasn't able to meet my grandfather, but

had heard he was a good, but strict man. Mom would tell

us stories of how he would whip them with "switches," which

were branches from a tree. He refused to put up with any nonsense. Maybe that's where Mom learned how to be strict. She loved to use a switch and would make us go outside and get one for her to use on us. For some reason, I would always be blamed for the actions of my younger brothers. I guess I was the oldest and was supposed to have been the one to keep a close eye on them.

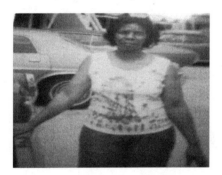

Everyone loved Grandma, especially her cooking. That's how my mom learned her skills in the kitchen. Thank God for Grandma Julia. When Grandma fell ill and was hospitalized it was hard on us. I remember, as a young child, going with my mom to visit her in the hospital. All children had to stay in the waiting room though. This was back in the day when children were not allowed on the hospital floors for fear of contracting some disease. Go figure. Grandma's health continued to fail, and it seemed as if she would never come back home. Grandma passed from complications secondary to diabetes. We were on our own. I hadn't seen her in so long. This was a difficult time for Mom and the family. It felt like there was a void in our lives. Who would we turn

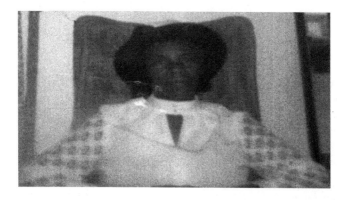

to when we needed help? I remember her home-going services as if it were yesterday. We were all packed into our family's church, the Sandy Grove Holiness Church, on a hot summer day. My youngest brother, Mario, didn't attend, but Terrance and I were there. Dressed in a white garment, the woman I called Grandma lay in a light blue coffin. This was the first time I'd seen her since she left home weeks prior to go into the hospital. It was a rough day for all of us, especially Mom.

Even in the midst of this, in the back of my mind, I always wondered where Dad was. He wasn't there when I learned to tie my shoes. He wasn't there when I learned to ride my first bike. He wasn't even there to see me off on my first day of kindergarten. *What a chump!* I thought. My dad had remarried and started a new family of his own. As we all know, with a new marriage comes new drama. I would visit my dad and his new family, and, of course, the conversation would always include my mom. For some reason, she was always portrayed as the "bad" person.

My dad would say, "Look at what you could have if you came to live with us." Children are impressionable. I wasn't exempt. I began to wonder why we had to struggle at home when my dad seemingly had the good life. He lived in a big brick home with a Jacuzzi on the patio, drove a nice car, and had cash to blow. "We'll build you a room," said my dad. My head had blown up so big, no one could tell me anything.

My mom began to notice that every time I went to visit my dad, when I came back home I had somewhat of an attitude or my demeanor had changed. She was correct in her observation. It would take me a while to get back to the real world. As I look back, I literally was being brain-washed. My dad was trying to convince me to leave my mom and come live with him and his new family. Whatever I needed, he provided. Whether it was shoes or clothes for school, I got it. Yes, I got it when I went to spend a few weeks with him during the summer or during holidays. It was odd that Mom always had problems receiving the child support check though. A mere $80 a month was my benefit for not having a choice in being brought into this crazy world.

The biggest drama was with my stepmother, of course. As a child, I never believed that she really cared for me. Maybe she thought I was taking my dad away from her or something. Most of my visits with my dad occurred during the summer months. My stepmother worked for the local high school and was off during the summer. He would give her money to take me shopping to purchase whatever I needed, within reason of course. I remember shopping trips to Myrtle Beach because there were no real places to shop in the city, Mullins, South Carolina, where my dad lived. This was a big deal, going to Myrtle Beach to shop. In the eyes of a kid, I had it made. At the time, he had three daughters of his own. Despite this, whenever I came around I felt like I was the prized child. He would take me to see my aunts and uncles, show me off at church and to his friends and say, "This is my boy." I guess I felt special. I received lots of attention. In the back of my mind, though, I would think about Mom and being with my real family. I didn't have to act fake around them. I didn't feel uncomfortable at home either. My smiles were real and genuine, not for show. When my mom complimented me or promised to buy me something, there was no hidden agenda.

For some odd reason, I never felt 100 percent comfortable being at my dad's place. I would limit the amount of food I ate. Even during dinner I wouldn't ask for seconds because I didn't want to be a bother. My sisters looked up to me though. This big brother thing was new to them and I guess exciting. I must say they were fun. Even though I had fun with them, I always felt that I was under surveillance by my stepmother. I'm sure that sounds funny, but I felt as if she was always watching my interaction with the girls. What would I do to harm them? I was their big brother. If anything, I would protect them from harm. I would be glad when Dad came in from work to help diffuse the situation.

My mom would call periodically to check up on me. This was the right, but wrong, thing to do. Cell phones were just appearing on the market, and most people who had money had the big, bulky bag phones. That would count us out. My mom had no choice but to call my dad's home number in order to speak with me. Boy, did Mom and his wife have some heated conversations over me. I think this is where I learned how to swear. The stepmom would ultimately get upset with Dad and would walk around with some chip on her shoulder. Of course, this made me terribly uncomfortable. Then, I knew it was about time for me to go home. Was I to blame for being brought into this world? I had no say so, but the arguments had me as the center of attention.

REFLECTIONS

What traits of the "settler" do you notice in yourself?

_____

_____

_____

_____

_____

_____

_____

_____

_____

_____

_____

_____

_____

_____

Chapter 1 Every Step

What parts of the "striver" do you see in yourself?

_____

_____

_____

_____

_____

_____

_____

_____

_____

_____

_____

_____

_____

_____

Overall, are you more of a "settler" or a "striver"? Why?

_____

_____

_____

_____

_____

_____

_____

_____

_____

_____

_____

_____

_____

_____

Chapter 1 Every Step

_____

_____

_____

_____

_____

_____

_____

_____

_____

_____

_____

_____

_____

_____

_____

_____

_____

Write about a childhood memory that molded you into
the type of person you are today.

_____

_____

_____

_____

_____

_____

_____

_____

_____

_____

_____

_____

_____

_____

Chapter 1 Every Step

_____

_____

_____

_____

_____

_____

_____

_____

_____

_____

_____

_____

_____

_____

_____

_____

Chapter 2
Keep Climbing

A s I grew older, I began to notice that my brother, Terrance, and I would be mistaken as twins. Even though we were a few years apart, people would tell my mom that she had such a handsome set of twins. It didn't help that she frequently dressed us alike. I wondered how this was possible since my dad refused to acknowledge him as his flesh and blood. Was it because we lived together in close quarters that we picked up

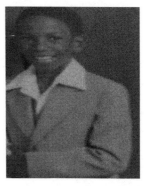 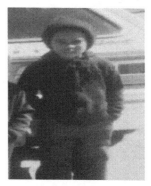

one another's traits and mannerisms? I was thoroughly confused and, at times, found myself angry. The anger surfaced as I thought about having to share everything my dad did for me with my younger brother. As I think about it now, I realize how selfish I was. I was a child, however, and didn't know any better. It was such a tangled web. It was not until years later that we would know the truth.

Sometime after Grandma passed, Mom moved us from the little town of Mullins, South Carolina to the big city of Columbia. There just were no opportunities for growth and advancement in that small town. Something had to change. We had to do something different.

"It may not be you, but your immediate environment that's hindering your forward progression."

"If what's in front of you looks like images in your rear view mirror, then you're headed in the wrong direction."

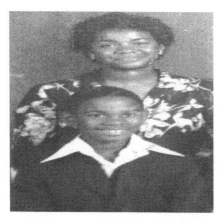

My mom worked extra hard to raise us, as would any strong, independent woman. I remember, all too vividly, when we each had three pairs of blue jeans to recycle and wear to school each week. "Didn't you wear those pants two days ago?" My response would be, "Yes, but they're clean."

Youth can be malicious at times, and often I felt quite embarrassed. My solace was the knowledge that my mother was doing the very best she could to provide the key things we needed. Yes, she was a single parent for most of my childhood. She knew how to make ends meet, even if it meant we had to go on public assistance and use food stamps. Back then, food stamps looked like paper money. No EBT card existed so there was no way to disguise it. I was mortified. We had to eat, but I hated going to the supermarket and having to use them. If my mom sent me to the store to purchase items, I would actually wait until the line was totally empty before going to the checkout counter. This was my way of protecting myself from embarrassment. It seems silly now, but when I was younger, it really bothered me. Though it may have taken me longer, it was worth it to preserve my sanity. Then there was the dreaded government cheese. This became a staple in our house, and we found ourselves looking forward to it.

For a certain period of time, we had no means of transportation, other than public transportation or our own two feet. I also struggled with this concept. I dreamed about my family doing more and having nicer things. We became accustomed to using the free clinic for medical care. My hat goes off to the Salvation Army and Associated Charities for making Christmas memorable. Despite the long lines and wait, we were able to get some great Christmas gifts. Now every Christmas, I make it a priority to visit the Salvation Army bell ringers to give a donation. Many times, Cooperative Ministries helped us keep our lights on. I appreciate what all the organizations did for us in our times of need. Thinking back on those stints makes me appreciate the present.

There was a period of time when we had to consider moving into public housing or as we called it, "the projects." Paying rent the conventional way and providing for three growing boys had become a strain. I'm sure there are many who can relate. This was one of the worst times in my life, or so I thought. A few months prior, we were considering moving into a nice brick home on the north side of the city. We visited the house, which was located in a nice, family-oriented neighborhood. It had nicer schools, nicer shopping, just about nicer everything. We were moving up. I was so excited. I had already made plans and could see myself living there. All of a sudden, it seemed like the world stopped for but a moment when my mom said that option was off the table, and we were approved to move into "the projects." Oh no, someone had to be playing a trick on me. Apparently, she had applied for public housing months prior and was placed on a waiting list until a space became available. I didn't know anything about this. I felt like I should have known. At least I could have prepared a bit better. I was devastated when, just before we were to settle into our new brick house, we received the call that said a space had opened up. The projects! The world as I knew it was over. I struggled for many months over this. I wanted to have the finer things in life, like some of my friends had. My mom had decided to go back to school later in life and was close to finishing her degree. I guess she felt this was the best decision for the family at the time. I'm able to understand now, but back then, I felt like my world had shattered. What would people say? How would I be viewed in the eyes of others? "There are bad kids in the projects," I told myself. Drugs, alcohol, noise, fighting were all the things I had associated with "project living." Little did I know then, that this would turn out to be one of the best moves of my life.

"We dream of the reward at the end of the journey.
Bear in mind that it's during the
process that we get our greatest
development."

"Never let where you come from determine where
you can go."

REFLECTIONS

Write about a time when you were disappointed.

_____

_____

_____

_____

_____

_____

_____

_____

_____

_____

_____

_____

_____

_____

_____

_____

_____

_____

_____

_____

_____

_____

_____

_____

_____

_____

_____

_____

How did you handle the disillusionment?

_____

_____

_____

_____

_____

_____

_____

_____

_____

_____

_____

_____

_____

_____

_____

_____

_____

_____

_____

_____

_____

_____

_____

_____

_____

_____

_____

_____

_____

_____

Chapter 2 Keep Climbing

What are things you should have done differently?

_____

_____

_____

_____

_____

_____

_____

_____

_____

_____

_____

_____

_____

_____

What good can you see now that you're able to look back with 20/20 hindsight?

_____

_____

_____

_____

_____

_____

_____

_____

_____

_____

_____

_____

_____

_____

Chapter 2 Keep Climbing

_____

_____

_____

_____

_____

_____

_____

_____

_____

_____

_____

_____

_____

_____

_____

_____

_____

Chapter 3
Almost to the Top

We moved to Saxon Homes, and, then later, to Allen Benedict Court ~ project living. The place was small, but big enough for the four of us. The walls were a bland cream color and the floors seemed like they were made of concrete. During the winter, they were so cold. "This isn't home," I thought, "This is just a temporary fix." The place felt drab with no personality. There were three bedrooms and one bath. Being the oldest, I had my own room; nonetheless, I still wasn't happy. Out back there was a makeshift clothesline. Most of us didn't have dryers at the time. The apartment walls were so hard that it was difficult to hang pictures or window treatments. The stove was a half-sized tiny one. I wondered, "Could this get any worse? We were there now, so we had no choice but to make it work.

I had my reservations about the kids in the

neighborhood, too. The good kids were mixed in with the not-so-good ones. I guess that's true in any neighborhood in America. There were "settlers" and "strivers." I chose to connect myself with the "strivers." Furthermore, my mother was strict with us, so we had no choice, but to do what was right. The schools were within walking distance. Soon, I became involved in after-school programs in the community and settled in quite nicely. In the back of my mind, however, I repeated, "I'm going to do better." I wanted a better life for my family and me. I remember one incident where my good friend, Tonya, and I were walking home from school, and as we said our goodbyes, I proceeded to enter my apartment. To my surprise, my mom had purchased a new microwave oven. I just knew we were "coming up" because, at the time, only those who were affluent had microwaves. I ran out the door and caught up with Tonya as she continued to walk home and said, "My mom went and bought a microwave." I don't know why, but I felt like bragging that day. It was like Christmas; my excitement was through the roof. That was the highlight of my day. I'm sure my friend thought I was talking about it too much.

Even though I wasn't totally pleased with living in public housing, it didn't stop me from excelling in school. Making the honor roll was common for me. There were both pros and cons to being a good student. The good far outweighed the bad though. Yes, I was called a "nerd." Sometimes I thought that was my real name. My frame was small, and I wasn't very athletic at all. I remember when I attempted to play sports; it only lasted about a week. Soccer just wasn't my thing. That was a challenge. I decided to stick to the books. Having said that, I believe the nerd stereotype fit me quite well. Nevertheless, my friends kept me grounded. My crew was Chris, Cindy, Robin, and Tonya. We all lived in public housing except Robin and Chris. We were a positive bunch, though. We went to high school games together, out to eat, and often hung out at each other's homes. We had lots in common. We were all "nerds." It's so important to fly with those who are going places. We all had aspirations of some-day going to college and becoming successful. We worked hard in school. So really, the name-calling didn't matter all

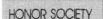
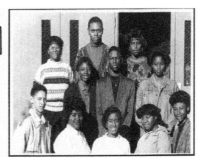

HONOR SOCIETY

left to right; 1st Row: John Kennedy, Rhonda Williams, Nichole Thompson, Robin Mazyck, Cynthia Linguard, 2nd Row: Miriam Cook, Rondrick Williamson, Tan-ya Dominick, 3rd Row: Yo-landa Nelson, Christopher Gladman, Joyce Williams

that much. Despite it, I focused on a much higher goal. It wasn't easy by any means, but I survived. By the end of my freshman year, I was used to it. People began to respect me for me because I didn't back down and let the struggle con-sume me; then, in the end I was victorious.

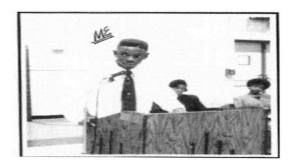

"Surround yourself with positive, motivating people. There's no room for pessimism or negativity."

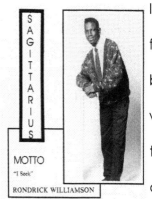

It's incredible how others ridiculed me for doing well and wanting to make a better life for myself. Interestingly, when I look back at those who were the main "bullies" to see where they are today...well I just won't say.

"Try not to be so angry with your haters. They just want to be where you are."

"When you judge and hate on others, it's just compensation for your own inadequacies."

I kept on doing me. It kind of felt good to be on the honor roll every eight weeks. The recognition was like fuel that ignited me to want to succeed even more. Keeping myself busy was important. JROTC, Drama Club, and Student Council were just a few of the ways I occupied my spare time.

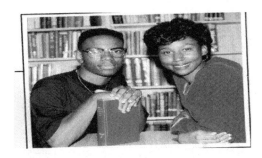

AFJROTC taught me the kind of self-discipline, self-confidence, and leadership skills that helped me successfully meet the challenges of adulthood. The program emphasized character development, leadership development, and community service. These were the same principles that my mom drilled into us at home. My first year in AFJROTC at CA Johnson High School, I was promoted to logistics officer. This was unheard of. I was only a freshman and already an officer. I could hear the grumblings from the upperclassmen. It was a great honor, though. This did wonders for my self-esteem. My high school years were a blast.

In my senior year, my classmates voted me *Most Likely to Succeed, Most Intellectual,* and *Most Dependable*. My close, dear friend, Cindy, won the same honors. The votes were counted, and there was no funny business. That year I pushed the envelope and ran for Mr. CA Johnson High

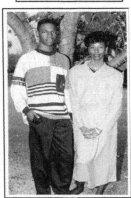

Senior Superlatives
Most Likely to Succeed

Cynthia Linguard
Rondrick Williamson

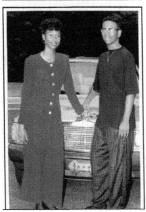

Most Dependable
Cindy Linguard — Rondrick Williamson

Chapter 3 Almost to the Top

School. That was totally out of my comfort zone, but it was

my senior year and I was trying to do something new. No

more nerd. I attempted to drop the old look and became

more "hip." I competed in an interview segment, a talent

portion, as well as formal and casual wear. Two of my close

friends were competing against me. The event opened with

a dance number that I actually helped choreograph. I was

a dancer back in my day. To my surprise, I won. It seems like

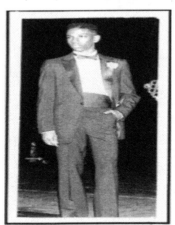

just yesterday I was sitting in my room rehearsing the dra-

matic monologue for the talent part of the competition. In

my head, I knew I was the best dressed in both the formal

and casual wear categories. I had so much support that evening. Of course, my mom and my brothers were there to cheer me on. They were my fan club. My dad and his family also showed up. It wasn't often that he attended any events that I participated in, but it was good to see him support this effort. I guess he had to start somewhere. The interaction between the two families was odd. Everyone was cordial

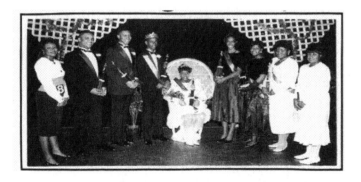

though. Having grown a bit, I was more aware of my parents' situation. Saying that it was a sensitive topic would be appropriate. Most of the time, it wasn't addressed, but as my maturity level increased, so did my curiosity. All of that was on the back burner that night though; I just wanted to wear my crown, take photos, and greet the audience. For the next year I would be on cloud nine. I was Mr. CA Johnson.

As the days of my high school years drew near a close, it was time to decide what to do next. Initially a career in the Air Force was number one on my list. For some reason, becoming an Aerospace Engineer appealed to me. I don't even know where the interest came from; perhaps I was drawn to it because the title sounded important. The Air Force was an idea, but I wasn't too sure. The only other via-

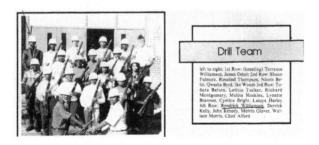

Drill Team

left to right: 1st Row: (kneeling) Terrance Williamson, James Odom 2nd Row: Shaun Fulmore, Rosalind Thompson, Nicole Belin, Qwesha Byrd, Ike Woods 3rd Row: Todara Belton, Letitia Tucker, Richard Montgomery, Melisa Hoskins, Lynette Brannon, Cynthia Bright, Latoya Harley 4th Row: Rondrick Williamson, Derrick Kelly, John Kenedy, Melvin Glover, Wallace Morris, Chief Alford

ble option was college, so I applied to keep my options open. All of my friends had high hopes of being accepted to a good college. Furman and Clemson University were my top picks. There were students from my high school who were attending these universities and gave rave reviews. These two schools had great academic reputations, too. Looking back, I really restricted myself by only applying to two colleges. The application fees were quite expensive so that limited my applications. What if I didn't get accepted? I prayed that at least one of them would want me. To my surprise, acceptance letters came from both universities. Clemson University was my choice. I received their letter first, and I was sold. This proved to be an excellent decision.

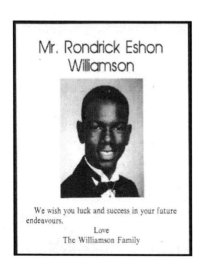

Mr. Rondrick Eshon Williamson

We wish you luck and success in your future endeavours.
Love
The Williamson Family

REFLECTIONS

Write about a time when what others thought or said about you affected your self-esteem.

_____

_____

_____

_____

_____

_____

_____

_____

_____

_____

_____

_____

_____

_____

_____

_____

_____

_____

_____

_____

_____

_____

_____

_____

_____

_____

_____

_____

_____

_____

Chapter 3 Almost to the Top

How did you overcome the stereotype?

_____

_____

_____

_____

_____

_____

_____

_____

_____

_____

_____

_____

_____

_____

_____

_____

_____

_____

_____

_____

_____

_____

_____

_____

_____

_____

_____

_____

_____

_____

What do you do today to keep yourself centered?

_____

_____

_____

_____

_____

_____

_____

_____

_____

_____

_____

_____

_____

_____

What do you say to yourself when you realize you are in a bad place and how do these thoughts help or hurt you?

_____

_____

_____

_____

_____

_____

_____

_____

_____

_____

_____

_____

_____

Chapter 4
Forward Progression

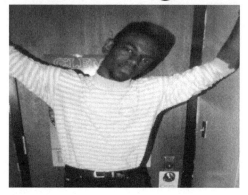

Going from a small inner-city high school to a large university was going to be quite a change. A tiger, I would be for the next four years. But what would I major in? That was the dilemma. Should I still pursue engineering? I don't think I was ever actually interested in it, but Clemson had one of the top engineering programs in the state. Decisions, decisions.

A shift occurred in my career path during the summer after I graduated from high school. One of the local hospitals, Richland Memorial, had begun a new summer program where graduating seniors could participate and get exposure to the medical field. This was an awesome new program. I needed another job. I was currently working at Food Lion after school and on the weekends as a bagger, and later, as a cashier. I submitted my application and was accepted. The program was from nine to four, Monday through Friday. That was just perfect. I could leave there and work a few hours at Food Lion in the evenings.

They placed me and a few others in the Radiation Oncology department. This department diagnosed and treated patients with cancer. What an experience. Not knowing much about medicine, I was exposed to patients who were battling this potentially life-threatening disease. The interaction with the physicians, nurses, and support staff was intriguing. Learning the process that patients go through during cancer treatments made me appreciate their struggle. They were survivors. Oftentimes, they were in better moods than I was. That was encouraging to see. The tide began to turn away from engineering to medicine.

With college, came great financial obligation. There was so much that needed to be done in preparation for Clemson. Of course, I needed luggage, a mini refrigerator, clothes, and so many other things. My mom was totally tapped out. With high school senior expenses, our limited income had taken a beating. In high school I wanted everything. There were letterman jackets, yearbooks, class rings, senior pictures, and the prom. The $95 registration fee for Clemson on-campus housing was due. We received this notice prior to my high school graduation with the stated deadline. Of course, I didn't have the funds and neither did my mother.

So, I called my dad. He said, "Send me the necessary information."

I forwarded him the materials and felt a weight lifted as I assumed he would take care of the registration. No worries, on to the next issue.

The time had come for new student orientation at Clemson. The college was about a three hour drive from Columbia. Our car wasn't in the best shape and also Mom couldn't take off work to make the trip. Because she wasn't able to attend, I tagged along with a fellow classmate who had been accepted as well. We headed up to Tiger Country. When I arrived on campus I fell in love with Clemson. There were tiger paws painted throughout the town. The landscape was filled with decorative flowers, shrubs, and fountains. The faculty and staff seemed genuinely friendly and inviting. I knew I had made the right choice. We went through the usual orientation lectures, registration for classes, campus tours, and signing up for housing. After waiting in the long line to see what my housing assignment was, to my amazement, I discovered that I had not even been registered.

What the what? How could that be? My dad was supposed to have taken care of that. I was embarrassed and afraid I might not have a place to live. Without housing, I wouldn't be able to attend. I felt my dreams slipping away. Only a few weeks remained before school started, and I had no place to live. The housing office said that all spaces were taken. My relationship with my dad wasn't the best, and this didn't make it any better. I don't recall ever discussing with him how inadequate this made me feel. Disappointed,

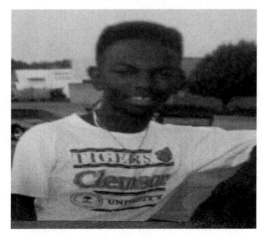

frustrated, and feeling helpless, I traveled back home to look at options. Would I have to postpone my college career until the spring semester? This plagued me for days. It seemed that there was no hope.

After speaking to the director of the summer program at the hospital, she said, "I have a close friend who works at Clemson. Maybe she can help." To make a long story short, I was able to be placed in a temporary dorm until a permanent space became available. The temporary housing situation lasted about three weeks, and then I was moved into a permanent space. Sometimes it's not what you know, but who you know that matters.

Don't let "set-backs" keep you from chasing your dreams. A "set-back" is just a "set-up" for a "come-back."

REFLECTIONS

Write about a time when you felt helpless.

_____

_____

_____

_____

_____

_____

_____

_____

_____

_____

_____

_____

_____

_____

_____

_____

_____

_____

_____

_____

_____

_____

_____

_____

_____

_____

_____

_____

_____

Chapter 4 Forward Progression

To whom did you turn to during these times?

_____

_____

_____

_____

_____

_____

_____

_____

_____

_____

_____

_____

_____

_____

What advice would you give to an eighteen year old starting college?

_____

_____

_____

_____

_____

_____

_____

_____

_____

_____

_____

_____

_____

_____

How can you apply that advice to your life today?

_____

_____

_____

_____

_____

_____

_____

_____

_____

_____

_____

_____

_____

_____

Chapter 5
What a View

After completing my summer program, college life was upon me. The staff and physicians from the hospital were excited to see me go and fulfill my dreams. Going from high school to college was culture shock, though. Having attended an all African-American high school, the racial diversity at the university was quite different for me. I didn't need too much time to adjust though. I could get along with anyone. It just seemed so exciting to be going to college. Meeting new friends, football games, pledging, and parties were all in the back of my mind. I guess the partying part didn't mean too much to me. I was never a party animal. I definitely did want to pledge a fraternity, though. Initially, I thought I wanted to join Kappa Alpha Psi. For some reason, they intrigued me. After taking some time to observe all of the Greek organizations on campus, I decided to pursue another–Alpha Phi

Alpha. It was a better fit for me. After a few months of set-

tling in, the homesickness went away. This was a process. I

missed home-cooked meals and having Mom do my laun-

dry. I wasn't ready for 100 percent independence but, inde-

pendence had begun. My character was developing.

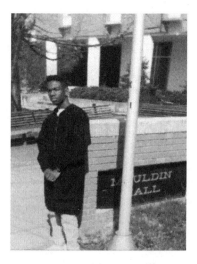

Even though I was away from home and in a new en-

vironment, there still was struggle. I did not receive a full ride

to college. Some of the expenses had to come out of pock-

et or from the dreaded student loans. When I went to the

campus bookstore to purchase my textbooks, I was floored. I

couldn't believe that a textbook could cost $200. That was

for only one book. There were about three to four more clas-

ses to go. We hadn't even considered other supplies yet.

Well, at least I wasn't alone. Other students were feeling

the financial woes of college too. Work Study helped pay

some of the bills; at least it provided the basic hygiene prod-

ucts and snacks. I chose the five day meal plan. That meant

I could eat at the dining hall five days a week. On the week-

ends, I had to provide for myself. Because of this, a great re-

lationship was established with microwavable meals.

In my mind, it feels like only yesterday that I was hiking

across campus from my dorm to Lehotsky Hall where I

worked in the Aquaculture, Fisheries, and Wildlife Depart-

ment. My chosen major was Biological Sciences so I as-

sumed that's why they placed me in this department. Never

did I want to study wildlife; I wanted to be a physician. The

experience was great though. My interaction with the pro-

fessors and staff in that department further developed my

communication skills. I am forever grateful to Rosemary and

Betsy who helped me with any problems I had. They helped make my college experience a nicer one.

Like most first-year college students, I wanted a car. That didn't happen. I was lucky enough to meet a few friends who let me tag along whenever I needed a ride somewhere. On the weekends, I would catch a ride home from some of my friends from high school. There were several upperclassmen at Clemson who had graduated from my area a few years prior. This made the transition a little easier because I knew a few people already. The relationships established at Clemson would follow me forever; however, my first semester was rough. Unlike many, I didn't develop "the freshman fifteen." My experience went in the opposite direction; I lost weight. College life took a bit of adjusting to. It was a whole new ball game, much different from high school. I only had fourteen credit hours. That was a light load compared to most of my friends who had eighteen to twenty-one credit hours. That semester, Inorganic Chemistry gave me a reality check. My grade wasn't as high as I wanted, but I passed. I didn't know why I struggled so much in that course. My way of studying had to change. The high school method simply didn't work anymore. I could only think back to freshman orientation when they said, "Look to your left

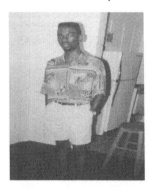

and to your right. One of these people won't be here after Christmas break." I was definitely returning by any means necessary. If it wasn't Inorganic Chemistry, then it was Biochemistry. This class was even worse. The Cooper Library became my closest friend. If I wasn't there, then I was shut up in my dorm room away from any possible distractions. I had to resort to audio taping the lectures and then transcribing them. When I started doing this, I began to see my grades improve tremendously. It's amazing that a class could be so challenging. If one scored between sixty and seventy on a test, they were doing well. Thank God for grading on a curve. These two courses were, perhaps, the most challenging of my college career.

Outside of the classroom, I found myself getting active in a few organizations on campus. I joined a mentoring group that paired freshmen with upperclassmen for guidance and direction. This helped a great deal. They shared personal stories about the classes and the professors who taught them. They steered us in the right direction as far as classes we should take to best suit our personal career goals. As freshman, we needed that type of peer mentorship. One of my classmates invited me out to Bible study one night and then to the campus Gospel Choir's rehearsal immediately after. Music was one of my first loves. I had sung in a few plays in high school and also in my church choir back home.

I ended up joining the Gospel Choir. Growing up, I would tag along with my mom to choir rehearsals. She was quite the singer. Most of her sisters and one brother sang. The family was full of "church singers." This is where I developed my love of music, especially gospel music. Every Sunday, it was a must that we attended church service. My brothers and I would sit back and watch as my mother sang with the choir. I sang with the Clemson University Gospel Choir for three years, and in my fourth year at Clemson I began directing the choir. We would travel locally and out of state to

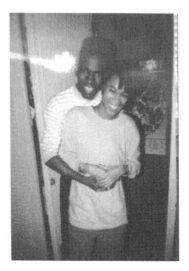

perform. Each semester we would produce a musical concert on campus. Tillman Hall would be filled to capacity with parents, faculty, staff, and fellow students.

During the summer months, I stayed on campus. I worked two jobs and took course work. Of course, my work study job was my main source of income, but I also worked as an Orientation Ambassador. We were responsible for campus tours and acted as hosts and representatives of the university during the summer orientation sessions. We were able to meet incoming students and also share our experiences as upperclassmen. Many of the new students looked up to us. It was easy to remember how lost and confused I felt during my first few weeks on campus.

I was able to complete the program and receive my degree from Clemson in exactly four years. In order to accomplish this, I had to take classes almost every summer. I was behind the ball because I only took fourteen credit hours my first semester of freshman year. I needed to catch up, and actually I looked forward to working and studying during the summer months. Because of this, my load during the regular year became easier for me to manage. The Bachelor of Science degree in Biological Sciences was well-deserved. It wasn't an easy task. I needed to figure out what my next step would be. Prior to graduating from Clemson, my medical school advisor introduced us to various career options for graduate school.

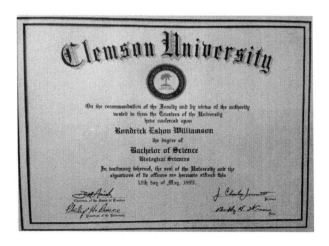

(

We considered allopathic medicine, chiropractic medicine, dentistry, optometry, and podiatry. Podiatry is what I chose, or I should say it chose me. Most people didn't even know what a podiatrist was.

It was commonly mistaken for a pediatrician. Nonetheless, I initially wanted to attend traditional medical school. I applied, as did many of my classmates, and for some reason my acceptance letters were slow to come in. I had my eye on the Medical University of South Carolina and Meharry Medical School in Tennessee. My application to the Ohio College of Podiatric Medicine in Cleveland, Ohio was submitted. Once again, I suffered through another game of waiting for acceptance letters to come in. Finally after studying and taking the MCAT exam twice, I received an acceptance letter from OCPM. It would have been devastating to get a rejection letter. When the letter came in the mail, I sat and opened it slowly. A rejection would have been the straw that broke the camel's back. Most of my other friends had already received their acceptance letters; so I was one of the few who were still waiting. Even though podiatry wasn't my first choice, eventually, I was notified that I had been accepted into the program, so I was determined to make the best out of it. After being accepted to OCPM, I began to visit podiatrist's offices to learn more about the profession. Some of the doctors didn't encourage me; some even made me second guess my decision. I was beginning to wonder if I had made the worst decision of my life. Even other physicians made negative comments about podiatry. At the time, podiatry just wasn't well-respected. My stress level was off the charts. I questioned my plans. Doubt began to enter in, and I found myself stressed out. It was a horrible feeling. Some of my friends and even some adults began to question my decision. They asked, "Why would you limit yourself by going to podiatry school? Don't you want to be a real doctor? Why work on feet all day?" I struggled with my decision. Was I making a horrible mistake? It was too late to turn back. The truth about podiatry would eventually surface.

REFLECTIONS

Write about a time when you began to doubt a decision you made.

Who or what made you doubt yourself?

_____

_____

_____

_____

_____

_____

_____

_____

_____

_____

_____

_____

_____

_____

How did you handle the stress?

_____

_____

_____

_____

_____

_____

_____

_____

_____

_____

_____

_____

_____

_____

Chapter 5 What a View

Are you now happy with the decision you ultimately made? Why or why not?

_____

_____

_____

_____

_____

_____

_____

_____

_____

_____

_____

_____

_____

_____

_____

_____

_____

_____

_____

_____

_____

_____

_____

_____

_____

_____

_____

_____

_____

_____

If you could go back and give yourself advice about this period in your life, what would you say?

_____

_____

_____

_____

_____

_____

_____

_____

_____

_____

_____

_____

_____

_____

Chapter 6
The Climb Continues

Before I could begin any medical school training, first I had to graduate from college. Graduation day at Clemson finally came. The day was full of joy and excitement. Because I was limited with only so many tickets for graduation, I only mailed invitations to a few family members. I did invite my dad and his family, and they

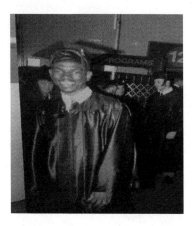

actually showed up. The day turned out awesome. No drama, no stress, just fun times. It wouldn't have mattered if no one had shown up but my mom and my brothers. They were my biggest supporters and, of course, a few other select family members who had always had my back. After the ceremony, we headed over to my on-campus apartment to gather my belongings. I said good-byes to my closest friends. My chapter at Clemson had

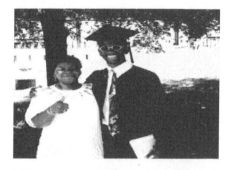

come to an end. What the future held in Cleveland was to be seen, but first we had to figure out how to get me there.

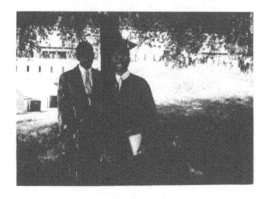

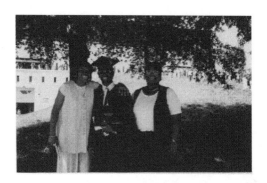

"Great things aren't accomplished overnight. It's a process. Surviving the process is our biggest challenge."

During the summer following my graduation, I worked hard to earn money to help offset the cost of medical school. My line of work was "cutting grass" with my uncles. Boy, did I hate being out in the sun all day, pushing a lawn mower, using a weed eater, and picking up paper. Summer days in South Carolina can be long and hot. I think I turned two shades darker that summer. At this point, it wasn't a choice for me, but a must. The expense associated with traveling to Cleveland for orientation and to find housing was great. So I labored in the field long and hard. There are some things I just had to do in order to get where I was trying to go. Little did I know; this was building and developing my character. So many people were counting on me. I would be the first doctor in the family. If that wasn't stressful, then I don't know what was. What if I failed to perform to the level needed to complete the program? I had already been given a warning by other podiatrists that I was basically making a bad decision. What a mess. My mom and family were proud of me, and it showed. How could I disappoint them? My dad began to tell everyone, "Meet my son, the doctor." Here we go again. I just would stand back and smile. The weight on my shoulders was heavy. It felt like a ton of bricks. To go to Cleveland and fail was unacceptable. The whole idea was so scary and uncertain. I would be about a twelve hour drive away from home. It wouldn't be so easy to swing by for a quick weekend visit. I'd never been that far away from my family and friends. I had no relatives in Cleveland. I would be out on my own. This was going to be interesting.

Did I back down from the challenge? No. Did I let the naysayers stop my drive? No.

"People want your harvest, but they fail to have seen the days and nights you labored in the field. Be careful what you ask for."

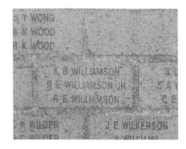
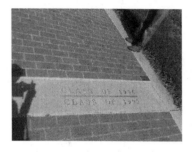

From early childhood to becoming a college graduate, I shared the most memorable experiences. What did I learn from those years of development? It didn't matter where or how I started, what mattered was where I ended up. In life, we will all experience times of turmoil and difficulty. These are not necessarily prescriptions for defeat. We often times need to change the way we look at things. The journey had definitely begun.

"Life has a way of strengthening us in and through our struggles and failures. Without failure, we often can't succeed."

The key to anything is finding a way to turn the negatives into positives. Be optimistic. It's a choice. Believing in yourself is most important.

"Never let anyone tell you that you can't accomplish what you've been destined to do. Follow your vision."

Sometimes we learn this the hard way. Would my life change tremendously going to medical school? The experience was quite like none other. This education thing was giving me a way of getting out of a tough situation. I had always imagined that a better life existed. Education would be the vehicle to take me there.

REFLECTIONS

Write about a time when you were afraid of failing.

_____

_____

_____

_____

_____

_____

_____

_____

_____

_____

_____

_____

_____

Chapter 6 The Climb Continues

_____

_____

_____

_____

_____

_____

_____

_____

_____

_____

_____

_____

_____

_____

_____

What worried you the most?

_____

_____

_____

_____

_____

_____

_____

_____

_____

_____

_____

_____

_____

_____

How did you handle the stress?

_____

_____

_____

_____

_____

_____

_____

_____

_____

_____

_____

_____

_____

_____

What have you learned from past trials that you can use to get through something that is worrying you right now?

_____

_____

_____

_____

_____

_____

_____

_____

_____

_____

_____

_____

_____

_____

About the Author

Dr. Ron is a physician, entrepreneur, mentor and motivational speaker. He has been featured on the daytime Emmy Award winning talk show 'The Doctors.' Other notable accolades include being featured in both Ebony and Shape magazines. Named as one of the 'Most Beautiful Doctors in America' in 2013, Dr. Rondrick Williamson literally built his entire career on hard-work and dedication to excellence. From humble beginnings, he has managed to create quite a presence in the world today.

He also has found time to pursue acting and entertainment, being coached by such greats as Terri J Vaughn, Cynthia Bailey, Tommy Ford and Rodney Perry. He has been booked for extra roles in VH1's Single Ladies, USA's Necessary Roughness, Tyler Perry's Madea's Witness Protection, BET's Reed Between the Lines, and most recently the Hunger Games: Catching

Fire. He has been featured on the Fobbs Business Review, Hilary's Hideaway Blog, the Ona Brown radio show and a host of others. Currently he is working on a major talk show project called, 'What the Doctor Ordered' with the Brook Entertainment Group in Beverly Hills, CA. He is also currently shooting the pilot for his own reality show, 'Dr. Ron- Unscripted.'

Dr. Ron can be contacted via:
Facebook: facebook.com/DrRondrickWilliamson
Instagram: thedrron
Twitter: twitter.com/ItsRondrick
Website: http://www.thedrron.com